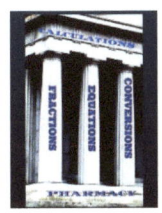

PILLARS OF PHARMACY

CALCULATIONS

FOR

THE TECHNICIAN

Vanessa LeSure-Walker, RPh

Author: Vanessa LeSure-Walker

www.theaphtiproject.com

The APhTI Project/ Vanessa Walker.—1st ed.
ISBN-13:   978-1514600344
ISBN-10:   151460034X

Tell Me, What Is Your Dream?

I could start by telling you who I am but I won't, not just yet. This book is about you! I know who you are, you are the person who wants to either become a pharmacy technician or you are **already a technician and you want to advance.**

That is why you are holding this book! You are holding the instrument of your next blessing...

You probably are at the point in life where you feel that it is too late for you to learn anything, especially math! You may feel ashamed to go back to school because of this weakness, your age or some obstacle that you feel is insurmountable--- but then there is that dream thing!

Your dream is what you see when you close your eyes at night! It is your dream that you make time to think of during the day! It is your dream that won't leave you alone!

Honestly, you won't be the best version of yourself until you have fulfilled your dream. There is more! You can't be the person that your children, spouse, nephew, niece, younger sibling... admire until you are your best YOU.

Your dream is something that you constantly desire to pursue but allow other things to get in your way! That madness stops right now!

Tell me what is your dream?

_____

_____

_____

_____

_____

_____

_____

_____

_____

_____

Why I am Qualified to Speak to You On This Topic

I am Vanessa LeSure-Walker! I am a Pharmacist by education and I have over seventeen years of behind the counter experience in both retail and hospital environments.

I am a Pharmacy Technician Educator and this is my gift, my calling is to teach. I have spent eleven years of my life teaching, training and developing Pharmacy Technicians and I have seen all types of students from the novice to the seasoned.

I am a self proclaimed Medication Safety Advocate, I teach people about their medicines and have written a book about that (it's called The TRUTH About What's In Your Medicine Cabinet). I go around and professionally speak about medication safety.

I love to speak about Pharmacy Calculations because I absolutely love to see the light bulb go off! There is a point where confusion becomes understanding and that is the moment that I look for in my students.

So as you go through this book, keep those things in mind.

I know that you know already, but write down your reason for wanting better math skills.

_____

_____

_____

_____

_____

_____

Let's Take Five

For some students, it takes one day and for others it takes one week. Different people process at different rates and most of that can't be changed. What the student can change is the amount of times he or she is exposed to the topic. In order to learn anything, you must increase your exposure to it. There is an old saying that Repetition is the Mother of Learning but I also have another, You cannot expect what you do not inspect.

So not only do you have to increase your exposure to the topic, you must do an inspection to make sure that you are on the right path to your desired outcome.

You wouldn't try to drive to California from New York on the first day behind the wheel of a car, would you? That would be silly, wouldn't it?

You also would not try to take the same trip without a roadmap or GPS or both, would you?

So why would you think that if you don't understand the math on the first, second or third try that it is useless and throw in the towel?

Remember your dream? If you stop because you feel that it can't be accomplished that is not good, let me explain why.

Unfulfilled dreams birth regret and the fear of trying something new. Your dream will gnaw at you one way or another. Either you have an anticipation of fulfilling it or you have the regret of not doing it. So either you look forward to accomplishment or you come down with a bad case of the dreaded "Woulda-shoulda-couldas".

One of my favorite singers, Kevin Lavar sings a song that has the lyrics of Procrastination being the mother of Regret. It is so true!

What am I saying? Understanding math is a process!

So let's proceed by doing an exercise.

Let's take five...

Take five minutes and list fifteen different ways that you use math on a daily basis. Ready, set, go!

1. _____
2. _____
3. _____
4. _____
5. _____
6. _____
7. _____
8. _____
9. _____
10. _____
11. _____
12. _____
13. _____
14. _____
15. _____

Did you get to fifteen? If not, find the closest person to you and ask them to help you with this exercise.

Let's Talk About Our Feelings

There is so much to know regarding math and the Pharmacy Technician. In order for you to be able to advance, math is one of the key elements that you are going to need in your quiver of arrows. If you do not have a good foundation in math, there is good news! You can develop it. It's like strengthening a muscle, the more you do it, the stronger and more proficient you will become. On the other side of the coin, if you don't use math regularly, you will lose the ability to perform even the simplest of calculations!

This reminds me of the time of my youth when I thought that I was not good in math and as I got older, I realized that I was fairly decent in math. Actually, it took an old classmate telling me a story about myself and math that I had long forgotten. This built my confidence! So when I teach my Pharmacy Technicians, I teach them from that vantage point.

But I remember as a child, in that moment, I did not feel that I had any math proficiency at all. Matter of fact, if you asked me back then, I probably would have said that math was not my favorite subject and definitely not my strongest one! What changed?

My feelings toward it changed! I started to see the value of a good math problem. I started to think of math's positive attributes. I love the fact that numbers do not lie (people do and some do so quite frequently)!

Why do I tell you this story? Well, you have to uncover your feelings about math if you want to grow in proficiency!

The reason why you *want* to become math proficient starts and ends with you! Yes, this sounds personal, doesn't it? Learning something new and different should be personal! Honestly, I have not come across a technician yet who did not want to advance. *Advancement* means different things to different people. To one person, it could mean a transition from retail pharmacy into hospital pharmacy. To another, it may mean remaining at a particular practice site, but being able to be paid more. To yet another, it may mean becoming the" go to person" in the pharmacy, an expert!

What does advancement mean to you? I am asking you seriously --- what does advancement mean to you? I want you to picture *how* you want to advance and write it down. This will be your reason why! In other words, when learning calculations gets tough, what is your why? What is that reason that is going to make you stick with it until you achieve proficiency? What is that reason that will make you put in the time to understand the math? What is you why?

_____

_____

_____

_____

If you are a Pharmacy Technician that understands mathematics, that puts you at an extreme advantage! When you want to branch out into the more advanced levels of pharmacy or you are in an advanced level and you want to get promoted, let's face it, math proficiency is one of those qualities that is very desirable.

One of the things that potential employers look at is math. I know of places that won't hire a technician unless he or she can pass a math assessment or is certified (and you have to understand math for certification to happen).

If the truth be told, I give entering students a math assessment before the enrollment process begins! This gives the student and me a barometer of where the student is, mathematically speaking and what we need to spend lots of time on in the program!

So tell me, what do you feel about math? If you like it, love it or can't stand it, just be honest! Then I want you to tell me why you feel the way you do and then (some of you will have to dig deep, I know) write one positive thing about math.

_____

_____

_____

_____

_____

_____

_____

The truth is, you need step by step guidance on how to perform calculations early on, especially if this is something that you have been deficient in the past. If you haven't performed math calculations well until this point, don't be disheartened! I am saying, "don't beat yourself up because so much of understanding and being proficient in this topic has to do with how you feel about it!" It is important that you start to get your mind right about the topic before you even begin to tackle it!

And another thing, you no longer have the luxury of telling anyone that you are bad in math! As a man thinketh, so is he---Proverbs 23:7. What you are allowed to say is something like this, " You know, I used to be weak in math but I am working on it and each and every day that I work on it, I become more proficient. I can even see the day when math problems will no longer be a problem for me!" How is that for a mood stimulating confidence builder?

Are You Ready For This?

I call this book, "The Pillars of Pharmacy Calculations", for a very good reason. A pillar is a structure that holds something else up. It is either a support or a monument. It is something upon which all else rests. I chose to call this article the Pillars of Pharmacy Calculations because there are some math topics that if you do not understand them, you will never become proficient. You may ask, what are these pillars? My response is the following:

- **Fractions**
- **Equations**
- **Conversions**

Visualize this...

 If you have just one pillar you have to make sure that it is centered and balance the object on top of it. If you have two pillars, it becomes a bit easier to balance your object and if you have three pillars, it is much easier to balance your object with some stability!

Before we delve into these topics, I have to say that you must make yourself understand the relationship of all of the characters on the stage. Think about the last time you went to see to see a movie or a play. You watched to see how each character interacted with the other characters and how they all acted in their environment, didn't you? Tell the truth!

Well, Pharmacy Math is no different. What I am saying to you is that in order to make sense of the math, you must thoroughly understand three relationships.

- *You must understand how each of the numbers relate to the other numbers in your calculation.*

- *You must understand how the numbers and the units relate to each other and, finally*

- *You must also understand how the units relate to each other.*

I have often heard students say that math looks like a whole bunch of numbers thrown together and because of this, math is hard to understand. The problem solver (you) must become engrossed in the problem. In order for it to become solvable, it has to become alive to you. It can't be static, it can't be boring. Problems are engaging and dynamic. It is your primary job to see them as so! Sometimes it helps if you can construct the story behind the problem, especially early on!

Know Your Limitations

There is more, whenever you use something, in order to be effective, you must know its limitations. Let me draw a parallel, You would not ask someone who has a problem with money to keep money for you, would you? I mean it would not be a rational thing to do. would it? By the same token, we don't measure weight with a graduate cylinder and we don't measure volume with a ruler. Any device or any method that you use has at least one limitation and you must know what that is in order to master its utilization. Having this knowledge gives you very keen insight. Your insight will lead you to mastery and your mastery will lead you to excellence! Keep this in mind because before this book is finished, I will allude to this principle again.

Your Reason For Getting It Right

Now, when we talk about calculations dealing with dosage, the whole reason for this is that we want to adhere to those rights of the patient. I am sure that we all remember the saying, "the right dose to the right patient at the right time..." So it is important to truly understand these rights. For instance if we dispense too little of a medication in many instances that could be just as harmful as giving too much! If the patient is under dosed, that does not help them manage the condition whether it be a long term disease or a short term one like an infection. Speaking of infections, if we under dose the patient, we run the risk of resistant strains of the organism being created, "superbugs", if you will. This is not a good scenario and is certainly one to be avoided.

On the other side of the coin, we don't want to overdose the patient either. This can cause all kinds of negative effects up to and including death. In some cases death is only the beginning----death because of negligence can result in lawsuits, higher insurance premiums and the list of negative results goes on and on.

Believe me, I am not telling you these things to scare you, quite the opposite. I am telling you these things to remind you of what is at stake. The reason why you *need* to become proficient at calculations starts and ends with the patient.

But do you remember me saying that the reason why you *want* to become math proficient starts and ends with you! Keep this in mind as we begin our process.

Let's get started...

Pillar 1—Fractions

If you struggle with calculations, the place where you need to begin is fractions, once you have a good handle on this topic, it will open up the doorway to understanding more complex calculations. When we talk about fractions we must know that a fraction is a mathematical relationship of division between or among two or more expressions. Very simply, at first we will say that these expressions are numbers but as we go on we will add more to this explanation. With fractions in their conventional form, there will be a number in the numerator and a number in the denominator. The numerator is the top number and the denominator is the bottom number.

$$\frac{numerator}{denominator}$$

We can say that the numerator is divided by the denominator or that the denominator is being divided into the numerator. In the case of 3/4, the numerator 3 is being sectioned into 4 equal parts. Once you have an understanding of this concept, we can then take a look at the types of fractions.

Whenever we see a relationship where the numerator is less than the denominator as is the case in

$$\frac{4}{5}$$

this is called a proper fraction. If we see a fraction where the numerator is equal to or greater than the denominator, we call that an improper fraction, as is the case with the following:

$$\frac{9}{7}$$

Improper fractions should always be converted into mixed numbers . An example of a mixed number is:

$$3\frac{2}{7}$$

Another thing that you must be aware of is that any number or value over itself is equal to one. So when the numerator and denominator are equal -- the result is one. This is another foundational topic that we must understand in order to do more advanced calculations. Dimensional Analysis (aka The Conversion Factor Method) uses this concept.

There are instances when we will have fractions in an unconventional form and when I say this I am speaking about decimals and percentages. Decimals look like the following:

0.16

4.2

0.088

Percentages look like:

45%

98%

100%

When we speak of percentage, it is understood that it is a fraction in which the denominator is always 100 and when we speak of decimals, the denominator is based on the place value of the last digit in the expression. For example, 0.9 means nine-tenths; 1.112 means one and one hundred twelve thousandths and so on.

If we have the number 24680.13579, the chart shows the values for each digit.

Ten thousands	Thousands	Hundreds	Tens	Ones		Tenths	Hundredths	Thousandths	Ten-thousandths	Hundred-thousandths
2	4	6	8	0	.	1	3	5	7	9

Numbers have no beginning and no end. There is no such thing as the smallest number and there is no such thing as the greatest number. The place value positions become as infinite as numbers are. This is signified by the line under the chart. The arrows signify infinity in both directions.

In order to understand decimals, you must understand place value . Since decimals and percentages are fractions, we must be able to convert our decimals and percentages into fractions and vice versa.

45%

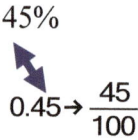

$0.45 \rightarrow \dfrac{45}{100}$

98%

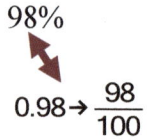

$0.98 \rightarrow \dfrac{98}{100}$

100%

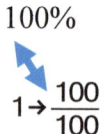

$1 \rightarrow \dfrac{100}{100}$

Now that you understand what a fraction is, the next step is understanding what operations involve them. While I know that we can add and subtract fractions, we won't go into that here. What we will focus on is multiplication and division of fractions. How do we multiply fractions?

The tried and true way is to multiply the numerators and get a final numerator then multiply the denominators, get a final denominator. Then place the final numerator over the final denominator and to get the fraction in its lowest terms, divide both the numerator and denominator by common factors if any exist .

For example:

$$\frac{3}{4} \times \frac{4}{9} = \frac{12}{36}$$

12 and 36 have the following factors in common:

1, 3, 4, 6, and 12.

So we will pick the highest factor that they have in common and divide both the numerator and the denominator by the same number. Since 12 is the highest, that is what we will use.

$$\frac{12 \div 12}{36 \div 12} = \frac{1}{3}$$

So ,

$$\frac{1}{3}$$

is my final answer.

This method absolutely works but it has one flaw. You must be able to isolate those factors that are in the final fraction. The issue is that the numbers may be larger than what you are accustomed to seeing and consequently common factors can be missed.

What if we could multiply and get as close as possible to our final answer and in the process increase our chances of getting the fraction in its simplest form right away? That would be fantastic, wouldn't it?

Well, this is the reason why we use the law of cancellation. The law of cancellation says that I can extract factors from the fractions before I multiply.

If there are common factors in a numerator and a denominator, I can divide each of those numbers by this common factor .

$$\frac{\cancel{2}^{1}}{\cancel{4}_{1}} \times \frac{\cancel{4}^{1}}{\cancel{9}_{3}} = \frac{1}{3}$$

When you really understand this, the concept that multiplication and division are the same process will become a part of your reality!

What do I mean? Well, let me illustrate this by an example. We know that one half of two is one or mathematically speaking

$$1/2 \times 2 = 1.$$

But isn't this the same as

2 divided by 2 is 1 $(2 \div 2 = 1)$?

Ok, not convinced, let's choose another set of numbers:

$45 \div 15 = 3$ and $45 \times 1/15 = 3$

This introduces the concept of reciprocals. A reciprocal of one number is the number that when multiplied by the original number the product is one. Mathematically, 1/2 and 2 are reciprocals because their product is one and 1/15 and 15 are reciprocals because their product is one.

There is a much simpler way of obtaining the reciprocal of a number. If we just flip the original number so that the original numerator becomes the denominator and the original denominator becomes the numerator, we can say that the original and the result are reciprocals of one another. See the relationships that follow:

2	$\dfrac{1}{2}$
5	$\dfrac{1}{5}$
1500	$\dfrac{1}{1500}$
875	$\dfrac{1}{875}$
$\dfrac{4}{21}$	$\dfrac{21}{4}$

Now, it's your turn, come up with three sets of reciprocals...

_____ and   _____

_____ and   _____

_____ and   _____

Pillar 2—Equations

Anytime we come across mathematical expressions that involve an equal sign, these expressions are known as equations. There are many times when equations can be used. For example, when converting between Fahrenheit and Celsius temperatures, we will use **9C=5F-160**. When we are doing a dilution we may use quantity times strength = quantity times strength.

I want to focus on another type of equation because without this equation type, many calculations become much more complex than they need to be. This type of equation is the proportion.

Proportions are used so very frequently in Pharmacy and I find them to be quite user friendly. In order to understand them thoroughly, you have to be able to see them and know what they are. Depending on how you look at them, you can say that they are:

a relationship of equality between two fractions, or

a relationship of division between two equations.

Look at the following example:

$$\frac{5}{9} = \frac{8}{x}$$

Here, we can either say that:

five equals eight when nine equals an unknown,

or

5 divided by nine equals eight divided by an unknown.

Both expressions are correct! The first expression highlights fractions with a relationship of equality and the second expression highlights one equation being divided by another.

To solve, we cross multiply:

$$5\,x = 9\,X8$$

$$5\,x = 72$$

At this point, we divide both sides of our equation by whatever our unknown is multiplied by, in this case the number 5.

$$\frac{5\,x}{5} = \frac{72}{5}$$

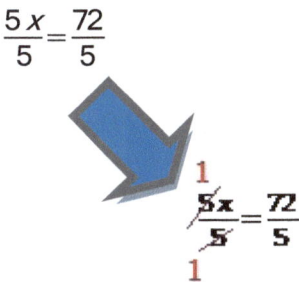

$$x = 14\frac{2}{5} = 14.4$$

If you have worked in Pharmacy for any length of time, you know that we don't just deal with numbers. We deal with units also and this point is illustrated in the next example:

A patient is to receive 400 mg of Amoxicillin Suspension. What you have in stock is a strength of 250 mg per 5 ml. How many ml of Amoxicillin is the patient taking per dose?

Knowing that the strength is stated as $\dfrac{250\,mg}{5\,ml}$ and our dose is 400 mg, we will set up our proportion like this:

$$\frac{250\,mg}{5\,ml} = \frac{400\,mg}{x}$$

Then we cross multiply (it is best if we temporarily drop our units to avoid confusion):

$$250\,x = 400(5)$$

then we divide both sides of our equation by 250, like this:

$$\frac{250\,x}{250} = \frac{400(5)}{250}$$

(I could have multiplied 400 x 5 and gotten 2000 but I wanted an opportunity   to cancel using the smallest numbers possible, so I am not likely to miss any factors.)

$$\frac{\overset{1}{\cancel{250}}x}{\underset{1}{\cancel{250}}} = \frac{\overset{8}{\cancel{400}}(\overset{1}{\cancel{5}})}{\underset{1}{\cancel{250}}}$$

x = 8

since our unit is ml, the answer is **8 ml.**

We must always express our units with their corresponding values. Placing our units into the equation, helps us, it does not hinder us. The positioning of our units tell us what to do if we are open enough to observe and take heed.

 In looking at the problem and paying special attention to the units, I know that my answer of 8 must be in ml. How do I know this? Aside from the fact that the question asks me for a volume. I know that 8 must be in ml because in a proportion, I must have two of each unit. If I look closely, I already have two numbers that are both in milligrams and there is only one number that is in milliliters. Therefore, my unknown must be in milliliters.

There are so many applications for the proportion! Proportions can be used for dosage calculation, for dilution problems, to solve for percentages, and the list goes on and on.

Pillar 3 —Conversions

In order to show excellence with calculations, we must know how to convert from one unit into another. Although proportions can be used to convert, they are limited. If there is not direct conversion from one unit into another, in order to use the proportion method, you will have to set up multiple proportions to arrive at the final answer. The more proportions that there are, the more likely that you will make an error.

Either you will omit something (you will forget to do something)or you will commit something (like rounding too early).

It is far better to use the method that I am about to show you. But first, I will work the following problem using the Proportion Method and then I will work the same problem using our next method, Dimensional Analysis.

Given the following problem:

A patient weighs 200 lbs, what is his weight in grams?

Suppose, you don't know the conversion between pounds and grams? Well knowing that there are 2.2 lbs in a kilogram and there are 1000 grams in a kilogram, you could set up the following proportions (fig 14):

$$\frac{2.2\,lbs}{kg} = \frac{200\,lbs}{x}$$

$$200 = 2.2x$$

$$\frac{200}{2.2} = \frac{2.2x}{2.2}$$

$$x = 90.90\,kg$$

then,

$$\frac{90.90\,kg}{y} = \frac{1\,kg}{1000\,g}$$

$$90909.09 = y$$

$$y = 90,909.1\,g$$

Remember when we talked about fractions and I said that any value over itself is equal to the number one? So any number over itself is equivalent to one, we know this.

Let me stretch your mind just a bit. Any two equivalent values over each other are equal to one. For example:

If

$$9-4=5$$

then

$$\frac{9-4}{5}=1$$

and the reciprocal is also true.

So if I know that 1000 g equals one kilogram and that there are 2.2 pounds in a kilogram, I can set up the following conversions:

$$\frac{1kg}{2.2lbs}=1 \quad \text{and} \quad \frac{2.2lbs}{1kg}=1$$

Since I am starting out with 200 lbs in my numerator, the conversion that I need must have lbs in the denominator, so that pounds can be cancelled.

Then I can work on getting rid of Kilograms and replacing that unit with grams which is the unit that I need. I will set up the following conversions with that goal in mind:

$$\frac{1000\,g}{1\,kg}=1 \quad \text{and} \quad \frac{1\,kg}{1000\,g}=1$$

Since Kilograms are in the numerator the conversion factor that I use must have kilograms in the denominator. So my full conversion looks like this:

$$(200\,lbs)\frac{(1\,kg)}{(2.2\,lbs)}\frac{(1000\,g)}{(1\,kg)}$$

Once the cancellation is done, the result is:

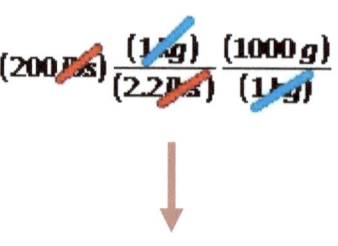

$$\frac{200,000}{2.2} = 90,909.09 = 90,909.1$$

Which would you prefer to do? If you are like me, you see the value in learning Dimensional Analysis.

Putting It All Together

Remember when I told you that doing math is like strengthening a muscle? In order to become great at the calculations, you must do them over and over again until you become strong.

These are the three pillars for calculations for the pharmacy technician. My goal in this book is to show the importance of calculations for the Pharmacy Technician and to show you how to use calculations effectively. In order for Pharmacy Technicians to advance, math skills are going to be needed more and more. Thank you for reading my book! I hope that I have helped you become a better technician.

About The Author

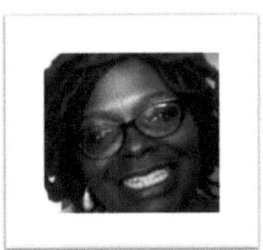

Vanessa_LeSure-Walker is a Pharmacist with over 17 years of experience behind the counter. She has worked in both Hospital and Retail Pharmacy environments. She has worked for over 11 years to help Pharmacy Technicians become certified.

She is the Founder of The APhTI Project and thus has taken on two very important missions. The first is to help Pharmacy Technicians achieve their personal best. She believes that in order for technicians to master all of pharmacy's moving parts, they have to be coached into it.

The other is to bring the topic of Medication Safety to the forefront of education. She believes herself to be a Medication Safety Advocate and encourages patients and caregivers to learn more about the medications that they take and/or administer. Vanessa speaks regularly on this topic and other topics that she is passionate about.

She has authored two other books, *The TRUTH About What's In Your Medicine Cabinet* (available on Amazon) and *Fundamental Formulas for Pharmacy Technicians*, a more comprehensive math book which will be released later in 2015.

She resides in the New York City area with her husband and two children.

For bookings and general contact, you can reach Vanessa at vw@aphti.com. Her social media information is as follows:

Vanessa Walker RPh

Facebook: facebook.com/theaphtiproject
Blog: theaphtiproject.blogspot.com
Youtube: http://bit.ly/16JGZtq
LinkedIn: https://www.linkedin.com/in/vanessalesurewalker